BECOMING THAT KYND OF PERSON

A WORKBOOK TO PROMOTE AND
INSPIRE PERSONAL DEVELOPMENT

BY KYLIE BRAGDON, ED.D.

BOOK COVER BY KYLIE BRAGDON
INTERIOR BY KYLIE BRAGDON

Dedicated to anyone who has needed a little help believing in themselves. This adventure in your development might be challenging, but I promise you are worth it.
~Kylie

Table of Contents

Introduction

I remember the first time I was told what kind of person I was, not knowing how significantly that moment would impact my future. It was a spring afternoon during my 8th grade year, and I was a quiet, naturally curious 14 year old who dreamt of big adventures. That day, my mom and I were scheduled to meet with the guidance counselor to sign up for my first high school classes, and this was an especially big moment for my family. I would soon be transitioning from a small coastal Maine grammar school of roughly 45 students to the larger community high school of 400. I was the oldest of two siblings, so we were in uncharted waters as a family unit, and much bigger waters than I was accustomed to.

To prepare for our meeting, my parents and I attended the "step-up night" at the high school. We met prospective teachers and listened to a presentation about the academic programs. I was immediately thrilled to hear about all the course options and was determined to take all of them, but a few slides later the idea of "tracking" was presented. To give you context, I attended high school in the early 2000s, and at the time in my community an emphasis had been placed on going to college. The school staff sold the idea like snake-oil salesmen, explaining that getting started on the right "track" early on would easily ensure your acceptance and future success in college. Given my experience at the open house, I was apprehensive entering the meeting with the guidance counselor. I weighed all of my course options and did my best to create a balanced schedule to include what I wanted and what I was told I "needed".

The counselor quickly reviewed my academic file as I handed over my list, nodding occasionally and agreeing with my selections. Things seemed to be going well, right up until we started talking about elective courses. Due to my rigorous course schedule, going into that meeting I knew I would only be able to fit in one "fun" course, and I desperately wanted to take welding. At the time, I enjoyed building things and working with my dad on his lobstering boat. In addition, I was already familiar with maintaining and repairing boat engines, and building lobster traps so the course seemed like a natural fit.

Boy, was I "wrong". Within moments of presenting the idea, the guidance counselor quickly explained that because I had straight A's and did well in science and math I really should focus on a college track. Her explanation, well "it would be more attractive to admissions offices" if I took a fine arts course. She further explained that I "wasn't the kind of person" that should take welding because it wouldn't be relatable to my future career. Overwhelmed by her feedback, I quickly complied and agreed to enroll in Introduction to Art for the first semester.

Though that meeting lasted less than 20 minutes, it left a lasting impression on me. I didn't take welding the next year, or any year of high school. Instead, I quickly conformed to the idea of who I thought I was supposed to be. This was especially easy because it seemed most people around me believed that I was the "kind of person" who went to college, whereas I, like most adolescents, wasn't so sure about who I was. Reassured by the idea that I was doing "the right thing", I pursued honors classes and varsity sports. I over-committed myself to clubs, volunteering opportunities, and social events, perpetually motivated by the idea that after graduation all of this work would pay off.

Spoiler alert, graduation came and went, and despite my many accomplishments I remained solely focused on doing the next "right thing". Like many, this vicious cycle of prioritizing what I "should do" over what I wanted to do continued through my early adulthood.

I pursued degrees, jobs, achievements, and relationships working tirelessly to be the kind of person everyone expected me to be. My "right" decisions eventually led me into an impossible job and a miserable marriage, both of which took a significant toll on my physical and mental health.

I had unknowingly treated my life as a checklist, but with every item I was able to cross off I sacrificed more and more of myself. It seemed like no matter how much I gave or how hard I tried it was never enough. As I neared a dangerous level of burnout, I realized I didn't want to be the kind of person that sacrifices their happiness any more, and through the desperate need to live life on my own terms the Kynd System was born.

If you have made it this far in the text, it is likely that you have also been impacted by the ideas society has imposed on you about what kind of person you are, leading you to make a series of personal sacrifices. At first it may have seemed inconsequential, trivial perhaps. Unfortunately, this type of thing has a horrible way of catching up with us, and the sum of those compromises has likely rendered your life unrecognizable. Thankfully, all hope is not lost. You can have the relationships, career, and lifestyle you have always imagined, the trick is to start unapologetically choosing you.

Before we go any further, it is important for you to understand what this book is and is not. This book is not a quick fix. It does not contain the key or universal "secret" to happiness. Instead, this book will teach you a system to fundamentally change your life through REALISTIC goal setting.

Beginning with a structured self-assessment, you will analyze each realm of your life to identify target areas for growth. After refining your goal setting skills, you will establish your short and long-term priorities so your personal development can begin IMMEDIATELY.

Supported by frequent opportunities for skill development and self-reflection, your personal development adventure will consist of five, 10-week cycles. During these cycles, you will learn how to set strategic bi-weekly goals and effectively track your progress. This new skill set will help you to gradually change all areas of your life, so that you can better live as the kind of person you want to be.

To support your development, this text will also incorporate an example character, Blake, to model how to use the Kynd System. In the "Relatable Skills" sections, Blake will also explore everyday challenges like all or nothing thinking, unrealistic expectations, and negative self-talk to demonstrate valuable strategies to keep you on track. Blake's examples will be highlighted in dark blue for your reference.

It is important to note that Blake does not represent a real person, but instead speaks to the generalities of the human experience. Many of these features were inspired by my current and past mentees. You may notice similarities in their behaviors, challenges, and possibly even goals. Despite these similarities, please know that this system is all about individualization. Your success during these cycles will be dependent on your ability to utilize the skills described in these pages so that you may consistently set and meet goals that fit your lifestyle, skill sets, and personality.

By moving forward in this text you are starting a new adventure. Inevitably challenges and obstacles will occur, however, consistent steps forward will lead to you changing your entire life. After completing the 5 cycles of this adventure, you will conduct a final reflection to measure just how far you have come. This is an opportunity to celebrate your major milestones and accomplishments, while also setting your eyes on what you will pursue next in living as your more authentic self.

So regardless of what you have been told by your family, friends, community, teachers or maybe even society, about what or who you are supposed to be, make the commitment to have this adventure on your terms.

Now it's time to ask yourself; ***what kind of person you want to be?***

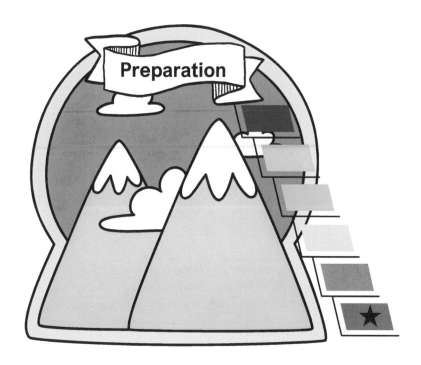

Preparation

What kind of person do you want to be? If you are still reading this, it is probable you fall into one of the following categories. You might be the kind of person who is unsure about who they want to be or what they want, but is desperate to make a change. If so, it is likely you have spent a large portion of your life doing what you thought you were "supposed to do " and have compromised your happiness along the way. Conversely, you might be the kind of person who knows exactly what they want, but can't ever seem to figure out how to get it. In the past you have probably tried changing different behaviors or aspects of your life, but your failed attempts have left you frustrated, angry, or maybe even hopeless. Regardless of the kind of person you are, the preparation phase of the Kynd System will help you develop the necessary knowledge and skills to support your long term success.

Self-Assessment

In order to effectively change your life, your actions must first have a deliberate direction. Unfortunately, life is not one-dimensional; therefore, finding direction can sometimes be challenging or overwhelming. To overcome this potential obstacle, the Kynd System identifies five major realms of life including physical, emotional, social, professional, and adventure. Each realm is described in greater detail in the area below, however; it is important to note this structure will be used throughout the text to help you organize and prioritize your development.

Physical: Related to your physical being and all the functions needed to achieve/sustain the lifestyle you desire. Includes, but not limited to, how you nourish your body, water intake, sleep habits, physical activity, and self-confidence.

Emotional: Related to what you think, how you feel, and how you interact with the world around you.

Social: All the areas of your life that prompt human connection. This could include, but is not limited to, your family, romantic relationships, friendships, community connections, and social interactions.

Professional: Related to your education, your employable skills, and how you contribute to society through paid and unpaid forms work.

Adventure: Includes your dreams for future travel, accomplishments, milestones, and experiences.

In the following section you will complete a short self-assessment for each of the five realms. This is an opportunity for you to honestly reflect on how you currently feel about and treat these areas of your life. Each section incorporates ten "I" statements that you will rank from "strongly agree" to "strongly disagree". The statements are meant to prompt you to think about your life critically, helping you to identify more specifically what changes you actually want to make. Upon completing each self-assessment there is an area for you to list your current priorities in each realm. Use this space to start outlining EXACTLY what you are hoping to achieve.

> To gain a more accurate understanding of your experience, it can be beneficial to complete one assessment at a time. Allow yourself the time and opportunity to complete an honest reflection, so you can confidently start you adventure in personal development.

Blake's Introduction

Blake is a 40 year old, married parent of two teenage children. Over the last fifteen years, they have prioritized the needs of the family and would largely be described in their community as "super-parent". Despite how others might see Blake, between their career, volunteering for the PTA, driving the kids to extracurriculars, and taking on the majority of household work they are just feeling an overwhelming sense of burnout. A recent doctor's visit also revealed a few health concerns that need to be addressed before they become a larger issue. In general, Blake feels tired, hopeless, and disconnected from their passions.

After completing the self-assessment, Blake identified the following changes they would like to make in their life. Review their results, then reflect on any similarities you may share with Blake in the area below.

Physical

- be more active
- improve health
- make better food choices

Emotional

- decrease stress
- do more things that bring me joy

Social

- spend more time with friends

Professional

- establish better work-life balance

Adventure

- be more spontaneous

Reflection

....
....
....
....
....

Physical: This area relates to your physical being and all the functions needed to achieve/sustain the lifestyle you desire. Includes, but not limited to, how you nourish your body, water intake, sleep habits, physical activity, and self-confidence.

	Strongly Disagree				Strongly Agree
I am typically well hydrated.	O	O	⊙	O	O
I regularly get enough sleep.	O	⊙	O	O	O
I eat a diverse and nutritious diet.	O	⊙	O	O	O
I do not over-consume caffeine.	O	O	O	O	⊙
I misuse drugs and alcohol.	⊙	O	O	O	O
I regularly engage in physical activity.	O	O	⊙	O	O
I do not have any mobility challenges.	O	O	O	O	⊙
I do not have any current health concerns.	O	⊙	O	O	O
I consistently take my medications as prescribed.	O	O	O	⊙	O
I am comfortable and confident in my body.	O	O	O	⊙	O

Reflection

In the following section, outline the changes you want to make to your body and how you treat it, to live more authentically.

....
....
....
....
....
....
....
....

Emotional: All aspects of your life that relate to what you think, how you feel, and how you interact with the world around you.

	Strongly Disagree				Strongly Agree
I can typically focus on tasks that require my attention.	O		◉		O
I consistently manage my time well.	O	◉	O		O
I feel positively about myself and the things that I do.	O		◉		O
I set boundaries to protect my emotional wellbeing.	O		◉		O
I regularly engage in activities that bring me joy.	O	◉	O		O
I easily manage my stress.	O	◉	O		O
I celebrate my achievements.	O	◉	O		O
I practice self-compassion during challenging moments.	O		◉		O
I am resilient to negative feedback.	O	◉	O		O
I am able to identify and prioritize my own needs.	O	◉	O		O

In the following section, outline the changes you want to make to your mind and how you treat it, to live more authentically.

....

....

....

....

....

....

....

Social: Includes all the areas of your life that prompt human connection. This includes your family, romantic relationships, friendships, community connections, and social interactions.

	Strongly Disagree				Strongly Agree
Generally, my social needs are met.	O	◉	O	O	O
I have a strong, encouraging support system.	O	◉	O	O	O
I am satisfied with my participation in social activities and events.	O	◉	O	O	O
I interact with my broader community in ways that interest me.	O	◉	O	O	O
I am happy and my needs are met in my current romantic and intimate relationships.	O	O	O	◉	O
I am content with my family structure and size.	O	O	O	O	◉
I feel accepted and included in my social groups.	O	O	O	◉	O
I have enough friends to share and pursue interests with.	O	O	◉	O	O
I am interested in pursuing new or alternative relationships.	O	◉	O	O	O

Reflection

In the following section, outline the changes you want to make to your relationships and social life, to live more authentically.

....

....

....

....

....

....

....

....

Professional: Related to your education, your employable skills, and how you contribute to society through paid and unpaid forms of work.

	Strongly Disagree				Strongly Agree
I have completed the necessary education to pursue the careers I want.	O	O	O	O	O
All of my professional training requirements are current.	O	O	O	O	O
I have secured the required certifications for my current position.	O	O	O	O	O
I am fully confident in my professional skills.	O	O	O	O	O
I am able to maintain a work-life balance.	O	O	O	O	O
I am interested in pursuing a different career or industry.	O	O	O	O	O
I am interested in pursuing a leadership role within my profession.	O	O	O	O	O
I am interested in sharing my professional skills through teaching or mentoring others.	O	O	O	O	O
I am interested in pursuing a position in a different organization.	O	O	O	O	O

In the following section, outline the changes you want to make to your professional life to live more authentically.

....

....

....

....

....

....

....

....

Adventure: Includes your dreams for future travel, accomplishments, milestones, and experiences.

	Strongly Disagree				Strongly Agree
I have regularly pursue my hobbies or interests.	O	O	O	O	O
I am satisfied with the amount I have traveled.	O	O	O	O	O
I routinely explore new places.	O	O	O	O	O
I am interested in learning a new skill or craft.	O	O	O	O	O
I am satisfied with how much I read.	O	O	O	O	O
I am interested in exploring new cultures	O	O	O	O	O
I would like to dedicate more time dedicated to creating art or a body of work.	O	O	O	O	O
I would like to learn more about a few topics I find interesting.	O	O	O	O	O
I have completed all the items on my "bucket list".	O	O	O	O	O

Reflection

In the following section, outline the adventures you want to pursue to live more authentically.

....

....

....

....

....

....

....

....

Self-Assessment Summary Sheet

Overall Ratings	No Change Needed				Significant Change Needed
Physical	O		O		O
Emotional	O		O		O
Social	O		O		O
Professional	O		O		O
Adventure	O		O		O

Identify three changes in your life that you would like to prioritize.

1)...

....

2)...

....

3)...

....

Identify three obstacles that have kept you from making these changes in the past.

1)...

....

2)...

....

3)...

....

Goal Setting

Congratulations! Upon completing the self-assessment you are one step closer to changing your life and securing a happier tomorrow. The insight you have obtained will be used in the following section, as we take action by setting clear and realistic goals.

By definition, a goal is anything in which you invest your ambition or effort.[1] They are a representation of what kind of person you want to be and what you hope to do. However, it is important to know that goals can occur on different scales. The larger milestones and achievements you want to experience are commonly referred to as macro-goals.[2] These goals are often associated with the big picture. Macro goals are the peaks of the mountains of your accomplishments. For instance, wanting to live a healthier lifestyle, securing a new job, or reading 100 books in a year are examples of macro goals. In contrast, micro goals are the steps you will need to take to make those larger macro goals a reality. For an individual hoping to live a healthier lifestyle, they might begin by setting a micro goal of walking a specific number of steps or eating fast food fewer times per week. The mountain in the image below symbolizes a macro-goal, whereas the steps represent micro-goals. Differentiating between these types of goals will help you establish short and long-term priorities.

Regardless of the type of goal you are setting, you can maximize the odds of your success by utilizing the S.M.A.R.T. Goal writing strategy. First introduced by George Doran in the early 1980's, this acronym describes the core features of effective goals. S.M.A.R.T. represents specific, measurable, attainable, relevant, and time-bound.[3] Each of these features is further described with examples in the area below to support your understanding.

Specific - This is a statement of exactly what you want to accomplish. Building on our previous example of the individual pursuing a healthier lifestyle, this statement might look like the following:

"I will walk...."

Notice how the statement is clear in who will be working on this goal and the action they will take.

Measurable - This is exactly how much you will be doing of the previously stated action. It is important to use a unit of measure that will support your success. For our previous example, this could mean measuring the amount of walking in steps, minutes, miles, or calories burnt. Whatever you select for a unit, make sure it is something you can easily and consistently measure. This feature allows us to expand our previous statement to:

"I will walk for 30 minutes....."

Achievable - When developing your goals, it is important to stay within your limitations. There are many factors including, but not limited to, time, money, and ability that may dictate your ability to follow through. While goal setting, it is vital to challenge yourself, but you don't want to set yourself up for failure. With this new information we can further expand on our previous example in the following way:

"I will walk for 30 minutes, 3 times....."

Relevant - When considering relevance, ask yourself, "Does this align with my overall macro goal?". Proceed with the micro goal only if it fits your original purpose.

Time-bound - This final feature provides you with a deadline for when you will complete the intended action. In the beginning phases of pursuing your, it might be beneficial to set shorter time frames so that you are encouraged to more regularly monitor your progress. We can now use this feature to finalize our example goal.

"I will walk for 30 minutes, 3 times by Sunday."

Though you might find it challenging at first, the S.M.A.R.T. structure will allow you to clearly outline each step of your adventure in personal development. As you begin this process, it might be beneficial to utilize the following goal template.

"I will _____ for _____, _____ by_____."

|(What you will do.)|(How much you will be doing.)|(How many times you will do it.)|(The day or date you will complete it by.)|

Macro vs. Micro Goal setting

After completing the self-assessment, it is obvious Blake needs to make some immediate changes. Given the outcomes of their most recent doctor's visit, they decided to prioritize addressing their physical and emotional realms. Before moving forward with any changes, Blake writes down a series of macro and micro goals, which are shown in the area below. Review the example, then take a moment to map out your first steps in your personal development adventure.

MACRO GOAL: *To live a healthier, better balanced life.*

MICRO GOALS:

I will walk for 20 minutes 2 times per week for 2 weeks

I will drink 80 oz of water 3 time per week for 2 weeks

I will practice self-care 3 times per week for 2 weeks.

Try using the following format when when setting your micro goals:
"**I will** _____ **for** _____, _____ **by** _____."

MACRO GOAL:

MICRO GOALS:

Challenges, Resources, and Timeline

Now that you better understand where you want your adventure in personal development to take you, it is likely you are feeling especially motivated to get started. Though we want to capitalize on this momentum, like all great adventures we must do a little planning. In the following section, we will explore potential challenges, resources, and timeline to ensure you have the necessary tools to be successful in meeting your goals.

Potential Challenges: This includes all external and internal factors that could disrupt your ability to meet your goal. External factors could include things like money, geography, time, personal support, or available community resources. In contrast, internal factors might include your time management skills, intrinsic motivation, or your confidence.

Resources: These are the tangible items, people, strategies, or structures you will need in place to meet your goals and overcome future challenges. In addition to identifying what you will need, it will also be helpful to identify if/how you will get those resources if you need them.

Timeline: Similar to your S.M.A.R.T. goals, when considering your personal development adventure it is valuable to develop a loose timeline. Begin by establishing an end date, which are often dictated by factors outside of our control. For instance, things like graduation, promotions, seasonal activities, and other opportunities may only occur during a specified time of year. After determining your end date, you can then develop milestones at the half and quarter marks of the timeline. As you progress in your development, you are encouraged to shift your timeline to better fit your needs as is necessary.

C.R.T. Outline

Prior to moving forward with their micro goals, Blake outline potential challenges, resources, and timeline in the area a below. This is the final phase of the preparation process and is meant to promote long term success by minimizing the impact of future obstacles. After reviewing the example take a moment to outline your own challenges, resources and timeline.

Blake's C.R.T

Challenges *Lack of time, not being able to disconnect from work, unwillingness to ask for help, feeling like i have to be "perfect"*

Resources *Help getting housework done from my family, boundaries for work, a more consistent schedule*

Timeline *Make health improvements before my next annual physical.*

Your C.R.T

Challenges ....
....
....

Resources ....
....
....

Timeline ....
....
....

Stepping Forward

The time has finally come to take action! You will be supported through five, 10-week periods of personal development. Bi-weekly you will to re-evaluate your goals and progress in order to better promote your progress in all realms of your life. Key features of the goal setting format are outlined in the area below. In addition, the following two week cycle example Blake's use of the structure for your reference.

A. Week Counter: Flexible timelines to help you document your change, regardless of when you start or if you take breaks between periods.

B. Realm Breakdowns: Color-coded to help you facilitate change in each area of your life.

C. Summary trackers: Allows you to reflect on your overall progress over the 2-week period.

D. Journaling Space: Areas to document progress, helping you to stay motivated.

E. Mindful Moments: Encouraging quotes and thoughtful statistics to keep you motivated.

F. Reflection Prompts: Consider key factors about your experience to promote your success in the following weeks.

Preparation

A. Week Counter: For best results, schedule a consistent day/time to reevaluate your goals each week.

Weeks 1 - 2

Physical

Goals: *Drink 48 oz water 3 times per week for 2 weeks*
Walk for 30 minutes, 3 times per week for 2 weeks

Summary Tracker

Progress

Drank 48+ oz of water Mon-Friday both weeks
Walked for 30 minutes Tues/Thursday both wek

Realm Breakdowns: This structure allows users to stay organized, and encourages them to set goals only in the relevant areas of their lives.

Emotional

Goals:

Summary Tracker

Progress

4

Social

Goals: *Spend 60 minutes with friends per week for 2 weeks*

....

....

....

Summary Tracker

Progress

Went to brunch with friends on Sunday.- 8/22

D. Journaling Space:
Track and celebrate your success in the progress sections. Record what you did and when on a weekly or daily basis!

C. Summary trackers: At the end of e
2-week period assess your overall succ
by placing an x on the scales. Remem
Blue=Your B

Summary Track

○ ○ **x**

Professional

Goals:...

Leave work by 5 pm 3 days per week for 2 weeks

....

Progress

Left work by 5 on Tues & Wed

....

E. Mindful Moments: Refer to these areas when you are in need of encouragement or further skill development.

Weeks 1- 2

Try using the following format when when setting your micro goals:
"I will _____ for _____, _____ by _____."

ADVENTURE

Goals:..
....
....
....

Summary Tracker

Progress
....
....
....
....
....
....
....
....
....
....

F. Reflection Prompts: At the end of each 2-week period, take some time to reflect so that you are able to better identify the next best steps in you adventure in personal development.

VICTORIES

1).......*Walked more than usual*.........
....
2).*Was able to drink water 5x week*.....
....
3)..*Didn't stay late at work everyday*...
....

CHALLENGES

1)............*Taking the time for me*...........
....
2)...*Saying no to extra tasks at work*.....
....
3)..
....

STRATEGIES FOR FUTURE SUCCESS

.......*Set up walking schedule for the week.*...........
....
....
....
....

In the following section, you will write your first bi-weekly micro-goals in the Phase 1 of your adventure in personal development. Please note, in the beginning it is especially important to promote your success by establishing attainable goals. These goals may first seem insignificant, even silly, but this immediate success will help you build confidence to face future challenges. As you make progress, be sure to document when and how much you accomplish. This information will help you to set more informed goals in the future. Finally, at the end of each period, you will complete a reflection on your experience to help you stay motivated and solution-focused.

As you move forward with your personal development adventure, it is important to understand that you will likely face obstacles and setbacks. You, however, get to decide the outcome of these challenges. I have complete confidence you are capable of any change you put your mind to, but please remember you are not in this alone! You can access additional support by joining The Kynd community Facebook group or by booking a 1:1 consult with me at www.thekynd.ca.

Now let's start becoming the KYND OF PERSON YOU WANT TO BE.

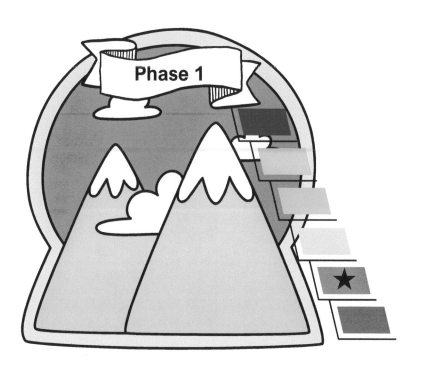

Physical

Goals:...
....
....
....

Summary Tracker

Progress

....
....
....
....
....
....
....
....
....
....
....

"Life is not measured by the number of breaths we take, but by the moments that take our breath away."
–Maya Angelou [4]

Emotional

Goals:...
....
....
....

Summary Tracker

Progress

....
....
....
....
....
....
....
....
....

Social

Goals:...
....
....
....

Progress

....
....
....
....
....
....
....
....
....

Professional

Goals:...
....
....
....

Summary Tracker

Progress

....
....
....
....
....
....
....
....
....

ADVENTURE

Goals:...
....
....
....

Summary Tracker

Progress

....
....
....
....
....
....
....
....
....

VICTORIES	CHALLENGES

1)...
....
2)...
....
3)...
....

1)...
....
2)...
....
3)...
....

STRATEGIES FOR FUTURE SUCCESS

....
....
....
....
....

Physical

Goals:..
....
....
....

Summary Tracker

Progress

....
....
....
....
....
....
....
....
....
....

Emotional

Goals:..
....
....
....

Summary Tracker

Progress

....
....
....
....
....
....
....
....

Social

Goals:..
....
....
....

Summary Tracker

Progress

....
....
....
....
....
....
....
....
....

Professional

Goals:..
....
....
....

Summary Tracker

Progress

....
....
....
....
....
....
....
....
....

ADVENTURE

Goals:..
....
....
....

Summary Tracker

Progress

....
....
....
....
....
....
....
....
....

VICTORIES

1)...
....
2)...
....
3)...
....

CHALLENGES

1)...
....
2)...
....
3)...
....

STRATEGIES FOR FUTURE SUCCESS

....
....
....
....

All of Nothing Thinking

In the past, Blake has tried some pretty extreme measures to reach their health and wellness goals. Unfortunately, Blake struggles to stick with these extreme shifts in behavior. To make matters worse, any time Blake varied from their original plan, they would perceive it as a failure and would immediately give up. If you have shared a similar experience, try interrupting this cycle of all or nothing thinking by initially setting goals that require little to no effort. For example, instead of setting a goal of going to the gym *everyday* Blake could initially set a goal of going two times per week. As their confidence improves, Blake will gradually increase the amount and/or frequency of their goals to further support their progress.

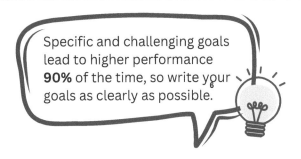

Specific and challenging goals lead to higher performance **90%** of the time, so write your goals as clearly as possible.

In the following area, identify goals that you have pursued in the past that have prompted "All or Nothing" thinking. Next, consider how you could rewrite that goal so it would require minimal effort for you to achieve in the beginnings weeks of your personal development adventure.

....

....

....

....

....

....

....

....

....

Physical

Goals:...
....
....
....

Summary Tracker

Progress

....
....
....
....
....
....
....
....
....
....

Emotional

Goals:...
....
....
....

Summary Tracker

Progress

....
....
....
....
....
....
....
....
....

"Success depends upon previous preparation, and without such preparation, there is sure to be failure." — Confucius [7]

Social

Goals:..
....
....
....

Summary Tracker

Progress
....
....
....
....
....
....
....
....
....

Professional

Goals:..
....
....
....

Summary Tracker

Progress
....
....
....
....
....
....
....
....

ADVENTURE

Goals:..
....
....
....

Summary Tracker

● ●   ● ●

Progress

....
....
....
....
....
....
....
....
....

VICTORIES

1)...
....
2)...
....
3)...
....

CHALLENGES

1)...
....
2)...
....
3)...
....

STRATEGIES FOR FUTURE SUCCESS

....
....
....
....
....

Physical

Goals:..
....
....
....

Summary Tracker

Progress

....
....
....
....
....
....
....
....
....
....

"I can do anything when I am in a tutu."
—Misty Copeland, [8]

Emotional

Goals:..
....
....
....

Summary Tracker

Progress

....
....
....
....
....
....
....
....
....

Social

Goals:...
....
....
....

Summary Tracker

Progress

....
....
....
....
....
....
....
....
....
....

Professional

Goals:...
....
....
....

Summary Tracker

Progress

....
....
....
....
....
....
....
....
....
....

ADVENTURE

Goals:...
....
....
....

Summary Tracker

Progress
....
....
....
....
....
....
....
....
....

VICTORIES

1)...
....
2)...
....
3)...
....

CHALLENGES

1)...
....
2)...
....
3)...
....

STRATEGIES FOR FUTURE SUCCESS

....
....
....
....
....

Consistency is Key

Blake has been putting in the work for about two months and is starting to notice improvements. Blake feels less out of breath when they go for walks and have more energy throughout the day. Though they are happy with the progress, Blake is finding challenging to stay consistent because their macro-goal of "Living a healthier, better balanced life", seems so far away. To overcome this obstacle, it can be beneficial to se a shorter term macro-goal for motivation. For instance, Blake might consider participating in a 5k or try to reach a PR at the gym. Frequently, the excitement of working toward a larger life milestone can help improve your focus and consistency. I

When individuals first experience failure when trying to meet their goals, **89%** of people will not choose challenges in the future.[9] Promote your long term success by setting smaller, more achievable goals in the beginning of your personal development journey.

What areas of your personal development are you having difficulty staying consistent? Brainstorm milestones you would be excited to pursue. Outline a timeline in the area below for meeting this goal and begin putting your plan to action!

....
....
....
....
....
....
....
....
....

Physical

Goals:...
....
....
....

Summary Tracker

Progress

....
....
....
....
....
....
....
....
....

Emotional

Goals:...
....
....
....

Summary Tracker

Progress

....
....
....
....
....
....
....
....

Social

Goals:...
....
....
....

Summary Tracker

Progress

....
....
....
....
....
....
....
....
....

Professional

Goals:...
....
....
....

Summary Tracker

Progress

....
....
....
....
....
....
....
....
....

ADVENTURE

Goals:...
....
....
....

Summary Tracker

Progress

....
....
....
....
....
....
....
....
....

VICTORIES

1)...
....
2)...
....
3)...
....

CHALLENGES

1)...
....
2)...
....
3)...
....

STRATEGIES FOR FUTURE SUCCESS

....
....
....
....
....

Phase 1 Summary Sheet

Rate your overall satisfaction with your status in each realm of your life.

Overall Ratings	Very Unsatisfied				Very Satisfied
Physical	O	O	O	O	O
Emotional	O	O	O	O	O
Social	O	O	O	O	O
Professional	O	O	O	O	O
Adventure	O	O	O	O	O

What three accomplishments are you most proud of during this period of change?

1)...
....
2)...
....
3)...
....

As you move into the next phase of your personal development, what three changes would you like to prioritize?

1)...
....
2)...
....
3)...
....

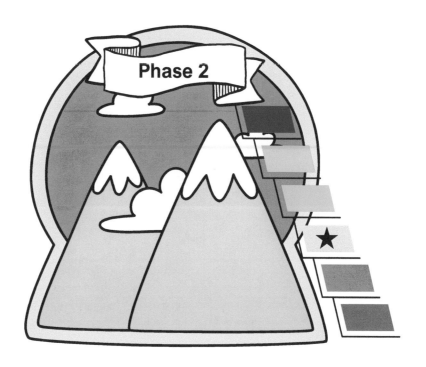

Physical

Goals:..
....
....
....

Summary Tracker

Progress

....
....
....
....
....
....
....
....
....

"If you have built castles in the air, your work need not be lost; that is where they should be. Now put the foundations under them."
– Henry David Thoreau 10

Emotional

Goals:..
....
....
....

Summary Tracker

Progress

....
....
....
....
....
....
....
....

Social

Goals:...
....
....
....

Progress

....
....
....
....
....
....
....
....
....

Summary Tracker

Professional

Goals:...
....
....
....

Progress

....
....
....
....
....
....
....
....
....

Summary Tracker

ADVENTURE

Goals:..
....
....
....

Summary Tracker

Progress

....
....
....
....
....
....
....
....
....

VICTORIES

1)..
....
2)..
....
3)..
....

CHALLENGES

1)..
....
2)..
....
3)..
....

STRATEGIES FOR FUTURE SUCCESS

....
....
....
....
....

Physical

Goals:...
....
....
....

Progress

....
....
....
....
....
....
....
....
....
....

Emotional

Goals:...
....
....
....

Summary Tracker

Progress

....
....
....
....
....
....
....
....
....

"Talent is cheaper than table salt. What separates the talented individual from the successful one is a lot of hard work."
— Stephen King 11

Social

Goals:..
....
....
....

Summary Tracker

Progress

....
....
....
....
....
....
....
....
....

Professional

Goals:..
....
....
....

Summary Tracker

Progress

....
....
....
....
....
....
....
....
....

ADVENTURE

Goals:...
....
....
....

Summary Tracker

Progress
....
....
....
....
....
....
....
....
....

VICTORIES

1)...
....
2)...
....
3)...
....

CHALLENGES

1)...
....
2)...
....
3)...
....

STRATEGIES FOR FUTURE SUCCESS

....
....
....
....
....

ear of Failure

ıke's commitment is finally paying off! They are walking regularly, increased their
ter intake, and has been more concenecious of what they are eating. More excitingly,
s is the longest Blake has ever been able to stick with a goal. Despite Blake's success,
ey can't help but be fearful of failure. In this kind of scenario, can be beneficial to
om out to re-examine your macro goals. Use a view of the big picture allow individuals
define key characteristics of what failure would look like and the reasons it could
cur. This information can then be used to proactively adopt behaviors or strategies
minimize the potential for negative outcomes. For example, when considering Blake's
ıcro-goal of "living a healthier, better balanced life", they determined failure could
ly occur if they gave up on pursuing their goals because they couldn't find enough
ıe. To help avoid these outcomes, Blake developed a schedule that they shared with
ɛir family so that they could have support staying on track.

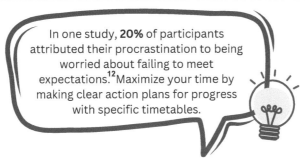

In one study, **20%** of participants attributed their procrastination to being worried about failing to meet expectations.[12] Maximize your time by making clear action plans for progress with specific timetables.

Identify key characteristics of how you define failure in the area below. Next,
strategies how to overcome factors that could prompt a negative outcome.
Begin employing these strategies *IMMEDIATELY* to help support our long term
success.

....
....
....
....
....
....
....

Physical

Goals:..
....
....
....

Summary Tracker

Progress

....
....
....
....
....
....
....
....
....
....

Emotional

Goals:..
....
....
....

Summary Tracker

Progress

....
....
....
....
....
....
....
....
....

Social

Goals:..
....
....
....

Summary Tracker

Progress

....
....
....
....
....
....
....
....
....

"I say if I'm beautiful. I say if I'm strong. You will not determine my story—I will."
—Amy Schumer [13]

Summary Tracker

Professional

Goals:..
....
....
....

Progress

....
....
....
....
....
....
....
....

ADVENTURE

Goals:..
....
....
....

Summary Tracker

Progress

....
....
....
....
....
....
....
....
....

VICTORIES

1)..
....
2)..
....
3)..
....

CHALLENGES

1)..
....
2)..
....
3)..
....

STRATEGIES FOR FUTURE SUCCESS

....
....
....
....
....

"I attribute my success to this: I never gave or took any excuse."
-Florence Nightingale [14]

Physical

Goals:..
....
....
....

Summary Tracker

Progress

....
....
....
....
....
....
....
....
....
....

Emotional

Goals:..
....
....
....

Summary Tracker

Progress

....
....
....
....
....
....
....
....
....

Social

Goals:...
....
....
....

Summary Tracker

Progress

....
....
....
....
....
....
....
....
....

Professional

Goals:...
....
....
....

Summary Tracker

Progress

....
....
....
....
....
....
....
....
....

ADVENTURE

Goals:..
....
....
....

Summary Tracker

Progress

....
....
....
....
....
....
....
....
....

VICTORIES

1)..
....
2)..
....
3)..
....

CHALLENGES

1)..
....
2)..
....
3)..
....

STRATEGIES FOR FUTURE SUCCESS

....
....
....
....
....

Avoiding Boredom

Blake has done a fantastic job sticking to their goals. Unfortunately, after completing nearly 4 months of the same workout, Blake is staring to get bored and is finding it challenging to follow through. To avoid losing momentum, it is valuable to pursue task that are progressively challenging. This could mean increasing the amount/intensity o specified goal or trying a new activity altogether. In Blake's scenario, to combat the boredom of walking 3 times per week, they could begin incorporating a group fitness class, running, or a strength training routine. Regardless of which option they pursue, this additional challenge is linked to their macro goal of "Living a health, better balanced life".

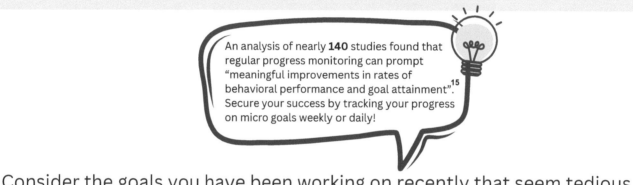

An analysis of nearly **140** studies found that regular progress monitoring can prompt "meaningful improvements in rates of behavioral performance and goal attainment".[15] Secure your success by tracking your progress on micro goals weekly or daily!

Consider the goals you have been working on recently that seem tedious or boring to complete. In the area below, identify ways that you could incorporate new challenges to help you stay motivated.

....

....

....

....

....

....

....

....

....

Physical

Goals:..
....
....
....

Summary Tracker

Progress

....
....
....
....
....
....
....
....
....

Emotional

Goals:..
....
....
....

Summary Tracker

Progress

....
....
....
....
....
....
....
....
....

Social

Goals:..
....
....
....

Summary Tracker

Progress

....
....
....
....
....
....
....
....
....

Professional

Goals:..
....
....
....

Summary Tracker

Progress

....
....
....
....
....
....
....
....
....

ADVENTURE

Goals:..
....
....
....

Summary Tracker

Progress

....
....
....
....
....
....
....
....
....

VICTORIES

1)..
....
2)..
....
3)..
....

CHALLENGES

1)..
....
2)..
....
3)..
....

STRATEGIES FOR FUTURE SUCCESS

....
....
....
....
....

Goal Summary

Rate your overall satisfaction with your status in each realm of your life.

Overall Ratings	Very Unsatisfied				Very Satisfied
Physical	O	O	O	O	O
Emotional	O	O	O	O	O
Social	O	O	O	O	O
Professional	O	O	O	O	O
Adventure	O	O	O	O	O

What three accomplishments are you most proud of during this period of change?

1)...
....
2)...
....
3)...
....

As you move into the next phase of your personal development, what three changes would you like to prioritize?

1)...
....
2)...
....
3)...
....

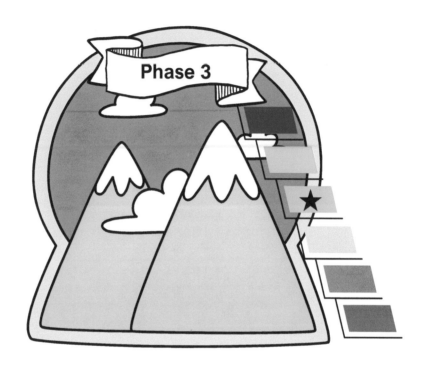

Phase 3

Physical

Goals:...
....
....
....

Summary Tracker

Progress
....
....
....
....
....
....
....
....
....

"It's harder to stay on top than it is to make the climb. Continue to seek new goals."
-Pat Summitt [16]

Emotional

Goals:...
....
....
....

Summary Tracker

Progress
....
....
....
....
....
....
....
....

Social

Goals:..
....
....
....

Progress

....
....
....
....
....
....
....
....
....

Professional

Goals:..
....
....
....

Summary Tracker

Progress

....
....
....
....
....
....
....
....
....

ADVENTURE

Goals:...
....
....
....

Summary Tracker

Progress

....
....
....
....
....
....
....
....
....

VICTORIES

1)...
....
2)...
....
3)...
....

CHALLENGES

1)...
....
2)...
....
3)...
....

STRATEGIES FOR FUTURE SUCCESS

....
....
....
....
....

Physical

Goals:...
....
....
....

Summary Tracker

Progress

....
....
....
....
....
....
....
....
....
....

Emotional

Goals:...
....
....
....

Summary Tracker

Progress

....
....
....
....
....
....
....
....
....

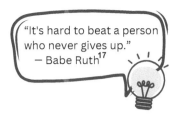

"It's hard to beat a person who never gives up."
— Babe Ruth[17]

Social

Goals:..
....
....
....

Summary Tracker

Progress

....
....
....
....
....
....
....
....
....

Professional

Goals:..
....
....
....

Summary Tracker

Progress

....
....
....
....
....
....
....
....
....

ADVENTURE

Goals:..
....
....
....

Summary Tracker

Progress
....
....
....
....
....
....
....
....
....

VICTORIES

1)...
....
2)...
....
3)...
....

CHALLENGES

1)...
....
2)...
....
3)...
....

STRATEGIES FOR FUTURE SUCCESS

....
....
....
....
....

Negative Self-Talk

After several months of consistent follow through, Blake has made significant progress in obtaining a healthier, better balanced life. Despite their gains Blake continues to feel like they aren't enough. When they fall short of their expectations even a little, Blake spirals into negative self-talk. This behavior impacts their confidence, and often makes them feel like giving up. To help overcome this behavior, it can be useful to write down the negative statements and then try to provide evidence of why these idea are false. This information can then be used to help restructure negative self talk into a more compassionate internal monolog. For example, Blake could restructure statements like "I suck" to things like "I am not where I want to be, but I am making progress".

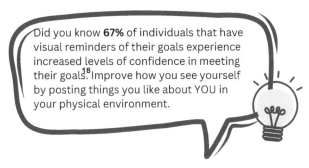

Did you know **67%** of individuals that have visual reminders of their goals experience increased levels of confidence in meeting their goals.[18] Improve how you see yourself by posting things you like about YOU in your physical environment.

In the area below, outline ways that you exhibit negative self talk. Try to then provide evidence of how these thoughts are not an accurate. Finally restructure the initial thought into a statement that is more self-compassionate.

....
....
....
....
....
....
....
....
....

Physical

Goals:..
....
....
....

Summary Tracker

Progress
....
....
....
....
....
....
....
....
....

Emotional

Goals:..
....
....
....

Summary Tracker

Progress
....
....
....
....
....
....
....
....
....

"Think like a queen. A queen is not afraid to fail. Failure is another stepping stone to greatness."
—Oprah[19]

Social

Goals:..
....
....
....

Summary Tracker

Progress

....
....
....
....
....
....
....
....
....

Professional

Goals:..
....
....
....

Summary Tracker

Progress

....
....
....
....
....
....
....
....
....

ADVENTURE

Goals:..
....
....
....

Summary Tracker

Progress
....
....
....
....
....
....
....
....
....

VICTORIES

1)...
....
2)...
....
3)...
....

CHALLENGES

1)...
....
2)...
....
3)...
....

STRATEGIES FOR FUTURE SUCCESS

....
....
....
....
....

Physical

Goals:...
....
....
....

Summary Tracker

Progress
....
....
....
....
....
....
....
....
....

"Take your victories, whatever they may be, cherish them, use them, but don't settle for them."
– Mia Hamm [20]

Emotional

Goals:...
....
....
....

Summary Tracker

Progress
....
....
....
....
....
....
....
....

Social

Goals:...
....
....
....

Progress

....
....
....
....
....
....
....
....
....

Professional

Goals:...
....
....
....

Summary Tracker

Progress

....
....
....
....
....
....
....
....
....

ADVENTURE

Goals:...
....
....
....

Summary Tracker

Progress
....
....
....
....
....
....
....
....
....

VICTORIES

1)...
....
2)...
....
3)...
....

CHALLENGES

1)...
....
2)...
....
3)...
....

STRATEGIES FOR FUTURE SUCCESS

....
....
....
....
....

Time Management

Recently, Blake's work life has been CRAZY! Staffing changes have required Blake to ta on a few new responsibilities, further increasing their mental load. Though they are trying to juggle it all, Blake finds themselves often over-committing time to some tasks while forgetting others altogether. To better promote their success, it will be beneficia for Blake to construct a more detailed day-to-day schedule. By setting and adhering to completing tasks at specified time, Blake can minimize the amount of wasted transitio time. This strategy also allows Blake to plan ahead so to minimize future stress and avoid missing deadlines.

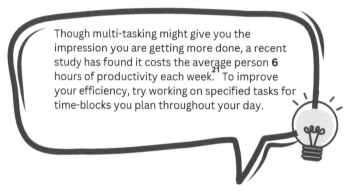

Though multi-tasking might give you the impression you are getting more done, a recent study has found it costs the average person **6** hours of productivity each week.[21] To improve your efficiency, try working on specified tasks for time-blocks you plan throughout your day.

In the area below, identify key tasks you need to complete in a typical day and the amount of time it will take you. Use this information to then map out your day in 15 or 30 minute increments. Be sure to include opportunities for breaks between major tasks!

....
....
....
....
....
....
....
....
....
....

Physical

Goals:...
....
....
....

Summary Tracker

Progress
....
....
....
....
....
....
....
....
....
....

Emotional

Goals:...
....
....
....

Summary Tracker

Progress
....
....
....
....
....
....
....
....

Social

Goals:..
....
....
....

Progress

....
....
....
....
....
....
....
....

Professional

Goals:..
....
....
....

Summary Tracker

Progress

....
....
....
....
....
....
....
....

ADVENTURE

Goals:...
....
....
....

Summary Tracker

Progress

....
....
....
....
....
....
....
....
....

VICTORIES

1)...
....
2)...
....
3)...
....

CHALLENGES

1)...
....
2)...
....
3)...
....

STRATEGIES FOR FUTURE SUCCESS

....
....
....
....
....

Goal Summary

Rate your overall satisfaction with your status in each realm of your life.

Overall Ratings	Very Unsatisfied				Very Satisfied
Physical	O	O	O	O	O
Emotional	O	O	O	O	O
Social	O	O	O	O	O
Professional	O	O	O	O	O
Adventure	O	O	O	O	O

What three accomplishments are you most proud of during this period of change?

1)..
....
2)..
....
3)..
....

As you move into the next phase of your personal development, what three changes would you like to prioritize?

1)..
....
2)..
....
3)..
....

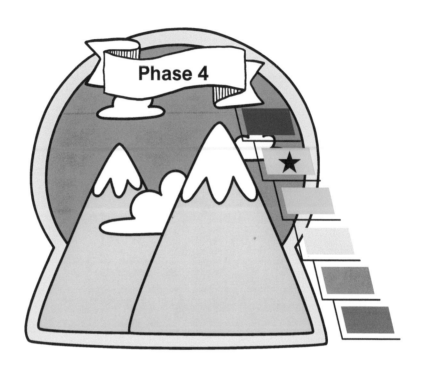

Physical

Goals:...
....
....
....

Summary Tracker

Progress
....
....
....
....
....
....
....
....
....

"Excellence is not a singular act but a habit. You are what you do repeatedly."
– Shaquille O'Neal [22]

Emotional

Goals:...
....
....
....

Summary Tracker

Progress
....
....
....
....
....
....
....
....

Social

Goals:...
....
....
....

Summary Tracker

Progress

....
....
....
....
....
....
....
....

Professional

Goals:...
....
....
....

Summary Tracker

Progress

....
....
....
....
....
....
....
....

ADVENTURE

Goals:..
....
....
....

Summary Tracker

Progress

....
....
....
....
....
....
....
....
....

VICTORIES	CHALLENGES
1)...	1)...
....	....
2)...	2)...
....	....
3)...	3)...
....	....

STRATEGIES FOR FUTURE SUCCESS

....
....
....
....

Physical

Goals:...
....
....
....

Summary Tracker

Progress

....
....
....
....
....
....
....
....
....
....

Emotional

Goals:...
....
....
....

Summary Tracker

Progress

....
....
....
....
....
....
....
....
....

93

"There is no limit to what we, as women, can accomplish."

—Michelle Obama [23]

Social

Goals:..
....
....
....

Summary Tracker

Progress

....
....
....
....
....
....
....
....
....

Professional

Goals:..
....
....
....

Summary Tracker

Progress

....
....
....
....
....
....
....
....
....

ADVENTURE

Goals:..
....
....
....

Summary Tracker

Progress

....
....
....
....
....
....
....
....
....

VICTORIES

1)...
....
2)...
....
3)...
....

CHALLENGES

1)...
....
2)...
....
3)...
....

STRATEGIES FOR FUTURE SUCCESS

....
....
....
....
....

Goal Sharing

Though Blake has remained fairly consistent, a recent change in their schedule has made it especially hard for them to prioritize their goals. At the end of most days they are feeling more tired than usual and it has started to effect follow through. When faced with new obstacles like this, individuals may find it useful can useful to share their goals with an accountability partner. For instance, Blake could share their weekly fitness goals with their partner, kids, or close friends. Frequently, individuals will be more motivated to complete their goals as they do not want to "let anyone down". In addition to improving overall follow through, accountability partner can also provide additional problem solve support as additional challenges arise.

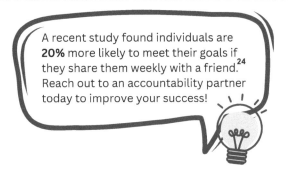

A recent study found individuals are **20%** more likely to meet their goals if they share them weekly with a friend.[24] Reach out to an accountability partner today to improve your success!

Consider what goals you could use additional support with. In the area below outline the what you are struggling to complete, who you will share your goal with, and how frequently you will check in to discuss your progress. Please note, you may want to consider using different accountability partners for different types of goals to better meet you needs.

, ...
....
....
....
....
....
....
....
....

Physical

Goals:..
....
....
....

Summary Tracker

Progress

....
....
....
....
....
....
....
....
....
....

Emotional

Goals:..
....
....
....

Summary Tracker

Progress

....
....
....
....
....
....
....
....
....

> "Don't spend time beating on a wall, hoping to transform it into a door." [25]
> - Coco Chanel

Social

Goals:..
....
....
....

Summary Tracker

Progress

....
....
....
....
....
....
....
....
....

Professional

Goals:..
....
....
....

Summary Tracker

Progress

....
....
....
....
....
....
....
....
....

ADVENTURE

Goals:..
....
....
....

Progress

....
....
....
....
....
....
....
....
....
....

VICTORIES

1)...
....
2)...
....
3)...
....

CHALLENGES

1)...
....
2)...
....
3)...
....

STRATEGIES FOR FUTURE SUCCESS

....
....
....
....
....

Physical

Goals:..
....
....
....

Summary Tracker

Progress

....
....
....
....
....
....
....
....
....

"You can't be that kid standing at the top of the waterslide, overthinking it. You have to go down the chute."
- Tina Fey [26]

Emotional

Goals:..
....
....
....

Summary Tracker

Progress

....
....
....
....
....
....
....
....

Social

Goals:...
....
....
....

Summary Tracker

Progress

....
....
....
....
....
....
....
....

Professional

Goals:...
....
....
....

Summary Tracker

Progress

....
....
....
....
....
....
....
....

ADVENTURE

Goals:...
....
....
....

Summary Tracker

Progress

....
....
....
....
....
....
....
....
....

VICTORIES

1)..
....
2)..
....
3)..
....

CHALLENGES

1)..
....
2)..
....
3)..
....

STRATEGIES FOR FUTURE SUCCESS

....
....
....
....
....

Overcoming Distractions

Lately, Blake has been feeling a little under the weather. With the recent change in seasons they seem to have less energy and are easily distracted when completing mundane tasks. In addition, Blake has noticed they have been mindlessly scrolling on social media or socializing with her colleagues at work A LOT lately. These distractions have begun to impact Blake's health and wellness goals as they have had to prioritize work task after hours. In this type of scenario, it is beneficial to establish more clearly defined structured work and break periods. To more effectively use this strategy, individuals should try to use their distractions (texting, social media, etc.) as a reward. For example, Blake could alternate between 45 minutes of work and then taking a 15 minute break.

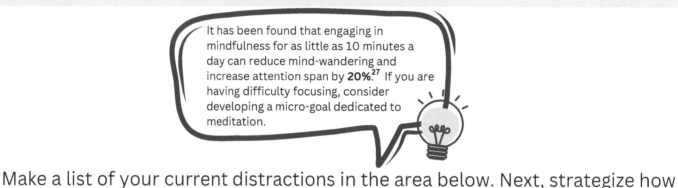

It has been found that engaging in mindfulness for as little as 10 minutes a day can reduce mind-wandering and increase attention span by **20%**.[27] If you are having difficulty focusing, consider developing a micro-goal dedicated to meditation.

Make a list of your current distractions in the area below. Next, strategize how you could use structured work periods to help you meet your current goals. As you continue to use this strategy, try to improve your work:break ratio to better fit your needs.

....
....
....
....
....
....
....
....
....

Physical

Goals:...
....
....
....

Summary Tracker

Progress
....
....
....
....
....
....
....
....
....
....

Emotional

Goals:...
....
....
....

Summary Tracker

Progress
....
....
....
....
....
....
....
....
....

Social

Goals:...

....

....

....

Progress

....

....

....

....

....

....

....

....

....

Professional

Goals:...

....

....

....

Summary Tracker

Progress

....

....

....

....

....

....

....

....

....

ADVENTURE

Goals:...
....
....
....

Summary Tracker

Progress
....
....
....
....
....
....
....
....
....

VICTORIES

1)...
....
2)...
....
3)...
....

CHALLENGES

1)...
....
2)...
....
3)...
....

STRATEGIES FOR FUTURE SUCCESS

....
....
....
....
....

Phase 4 Summary

Rate your overall satisfaction with your status in each realm of your life.

Overall Ratings	Very Unsatisfied				Very Satisfied
Physical	O	O	O	O	O
Emotional	O	O	O	O	O
Social	O	O	O	O	O
Professional	O	O	O	O	O
Adventure	O	O	O	O	O

What three accomplishments are you most proud of during this period of change?

1)...
....
2)...
....
3)...
....

As you move into the next phase of your personal development, what three changes would you like to prioritize?

1)...
....
2)...
....
3)...
....

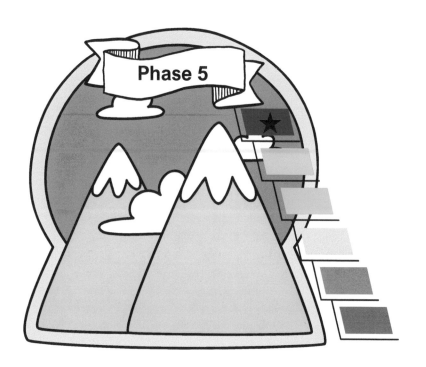

Physical

Goals:...
....
....
....

Summary Tracker

Progress

....
....
....
....
....
....
....
....
....
....

"You can always find a
solution if you try hard
enough." 28
- Lori Greiner

Emotional

Goals:...
....
....
....

Summary Tracker

Progress

....
....
....
....
....
....
....
....
....

Social

Goals:...
....
....
....

Progress

....
....
....
....
....
....
....
....
....

Professional

Goals:...
....
....
....

Progress

....
....
....
....
....
....
....
....

ADVENTURE

Goals:..
....
....
....

Summary Tracker

Progress

....
....
....
....
....
....
....
....
....
....

VICTORIES

1)..
....
2)..
....
3)..
....

CHALLENGES

1)..
....
2)..
....
3)..
....

STRATEGIES FOR FUTURE SUCCESS

....
....
....
....
....

Physical

Goals:...
....
....
....

Summary Tracker

Progress

....
....
....
....
....
....
....
....
....
....

Emotional

Goals:...
....
....
....

Summary Tracker

Progress

....
....
....
....
....
....
....
....
....

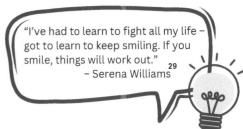

"I've had to learn to fight all my life – got to learn to keep smiling. If you smile, things will work out." [29]
– Serena Williams

Social

Goals:...
....
....
....

Summary Tracker

Progress

....
....
....
....
....
....
....
....
....

Professional

Goals:...
....
....
....

Summary Tracker

Progress

....
....
....
....
....
....
....
....
....

ADVENTURE

Goals:..
....
....
....

Summary Tracker

Progress

....
....
....
....
....
....
....
....
....
....

VICTORIES

1)...
....
2)...
....
3)...
....

CHALLENGES

1)...
....
2)...
....
3)...
....

STRATEGIES FOR FUTURE SUCCESS

....
....
....
....
....

Self-Advocacy

As Blake shifted their priorities to practicing better self-care and wellness, they noticed they are often forced to pick between *what they wanted to do* and what they felt like *they had to do* to help others. Though Blake customarily has taken on a lot of extra household or work tasks, they simply didn't have enough time to do it all. To address this challenge, it is necessary to self-advocate for additional support. Individuals should begin by creating a list of tasks they are responsible for, so they can more easily communicate their needs. Delegating small tasks a few times per week can dramatically impact the amount of available time. For instance, Blake typically does the dishes after dinner. If their partner took on this task three times per week, it would give Blake enough time to fit in their fitness plan.

if you struggle with self-advocacy, it is important to know you aren't alone. In one study, it was found 45% of women do not advocate enough or AT ALL.[30] Overcome this challenge by making self-advocacy part of your weekly or bi-weekly routine.

In the area below, outline tasks that you could use support with. Consider who could help you and how frequently they would need to complete the task to allow you to better meet your goals. **Now go SELF-ADVOCATE!**

....
....
....
....
....
....
....
....
....

Physical

Goals:..
....
....
....

Progress
....
....
....
....
....
....
....
....
....
....

Emotional

Goals:..
....
....
....

Progress
....
....
....
....
....
....
....
....

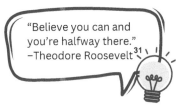

"Believe you can and you're halfway there."
–Theodore Roosevelt[31]

Social

Goals:..
....
....
....

Summary Tracker

Progress
....
....
....
....
....
....
....
....
....

Professional

Goals:..
....
....
....

Summary Tracker

Progress
....
....
....
....
....
....
....
....
....

ADVENTURE

Goals:..
....
....
....

Summary Tracker

Progress

....
....
....
....
....
....
....
....
....

VICTORIES

1)...
....
2)...
....
3)...
....

CHALLENGES

1)...
....
2)...
....
3)...
....

STRATEGIES FOR FUTURE SUCCESS

....
....
....
....
....

Physical

Goals:..
....
....
....

Summary Tracker

Progress

....
....
....
....
....
....
....
....
....
....

"I'm a success today because I had a friend who believed in me and I didn't have the heart to let him down." [32]
— Abraham Lincoln

Emotional

Goals:..
....
....
....

Summary Tracker

Progress

....
....
....
....
....
....
....
....
....

Social

Goals:...
....
....
....

Summary Tracker

Progress

....
....
....
....
....
....
....
....
....

Professional

Goals:...
....
....
....

Summary Tracker

Progress

....
....
....
....
....
....
....
....
....

ADVENTURE

Goals:..
....
....
....

Summary Tracker

Progress

....
....
....
....
....
....
....
....
....

VICTORIES

1)...
....
2)...
....
3)...
....

CHALLENGES

1)...
....
2)...
....
3)...
....

STRATEGIES FOR FUTURE SUCCESS

....
....
....
....

Scaling up

Blake has dedicated over 10 months pursuing their macro-goal of living a healthier, better balanced life. During this time they have learned how to prioritize and advocate for their needs, as well as improved their health and overall fitness. Blake no longer feeling an overwhelming sense of burnout and has accomplished things they never imagined possible. To continue to promote their personal development, now is an invaluable time for Blake to consider how they would to continue their adventure. Proactive planning for future milestones can help individuals avoid slipping into form bad habits and maintain focus. In this time in Blakes journey, they might consider expanding on their fitness goals to participate in a fundraising 10k or pursue a new outdoor activity to help stay motivated.

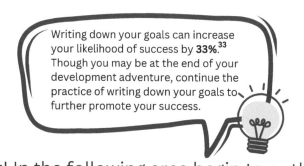

Writing down your goals can increase your likelihood of success by **33%**.[33] Though you may be at the end of your development adventure, continue the practice of writing down your goals to further promote your success.

The sky is the limit! In the following area begin to outline how you might continue your personal development. What crazy idea will spur your next big adventure?

....

....

....

....

....

....

....

....

....

....

Physical

Goals:...
....
....
....

Summary Tracker

Progress

....
....
....
....
....
....
....
....
....

Emotional

Goals:...
....
....
....

Summary Tracker

Progress

....
....
....
....
....
....
....
....

Social

Goals:..
....
....

Summary Tracker

....

Progress

....
....
....
....
....
....
....
....
....

Professional

Goals:..
....
....

Summary Tracker

....

Progress

....
....
....
....
....
....
....
....

ADVENTURE

Goals:..
....
....
....

Summary Tracker

Progress

....
....
....
....
....
....
....
....
....

VICTORIES	CHALLENGES

1)..
....
2)..
....
3)..
....

1)...
....
2)...
....
3)...

STRATEGIES FOR FUTURE SUCCESS

....
....
....
....
....

Rate your overall satisfaction with your status in each realm of your life.

Overall Ratings	Very Unsatisfied				Very Satisfied
Physical	O	O	O	O	O
Emotional	O	O	O	O	O
Social	O	O	O	O	O
Professional	O	O	O	O	O
Adventure	O	O	O	O	O

What three accomplishments are you most of proud during this period of change?

1)..
....
2)..
....
3)..
....

As you move into the next phase of your personal development, what three changes would you like to prioritize?

1)..
....
2)..
....
3)..
....

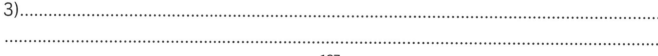

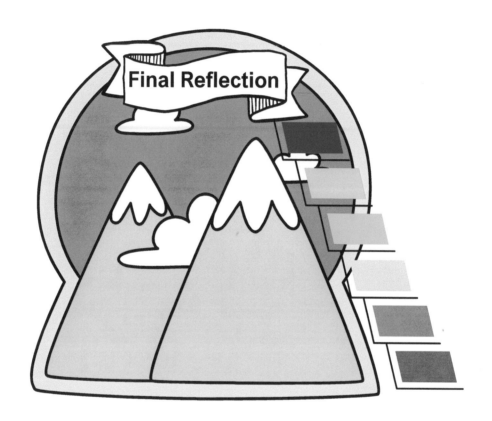

Final Reflection

Final Reflection

Congratulations, you have completed 50 weeks of personal development! With the support of this text, your consistent and strategic goal setting has empowered you to radically change your life. Perhaps more importantly, I hope this process has shown you that regardless of your situation you are **CAPABLE** of becoming the Kynd of person you want to be.

To understand the breadth of your transformation, the original self-assessment from the preparation phase has been included below. Take a moment to reassess your progress and highlight your accomplishments. You now have the skills to use this reflection to help guide your direction as you continue your adventure in personal development. I wish you the greatest luck as you continue to redefine and live as your authentic self.

Physical				
	Strongly Disagree			Strongly Agree
I am typically well hydrated.	O	O	O	O	O
I regularly get enough sleep.	O	O	O	O	O
I eat a diverse and nutritious diet.	O	O	O	O	O
I do not over-consume caffeine.	O	O	O	O	O
I misuse drugs and alcohol.	O	O	O	O	O
I regularly engage in physical activity.	O	O	O	O	O
I do not have any mobility challenges.	O	O	O	O	O
I do not have any current health concerns.	O	O	O	O	O
I consistently take my medications as prescribed.	O	O	O	O	O
I am comfortable and confident in my body.	O	O	O	O	O

Emotional

	Strongly Disagree				Strongly Agree
I can typically focus on tasks that require my attention.	O	O	O	O	O
I consistently manage my time well.	O	O	O	O	O
I feel positively about myself and the things that I do.	O	O	O	O	O
I set boundaries to protect my emotional wellbeing.	O		O	O	O
I regularly engage in activities that bring me joy.	O	O	O	O	O
I easily manage my stress.	O	O	O	O	O
I celebrate my achievements.	O	O	O	O	O
I practice self-compassion during challenging moments.	O	O	O	O	O
I am resilient to negative feedback.	O	O	O	O	O
I am able to identify and prioritize my own needs.	O	O	O	O	O

Social

	Strongly Disagree				Strongly Agree
Generally, my social needs are met.	O	O	O		O
I have a strong, encouraging support system.	O	O	O		O
I am satisfied with my participation in social activities and events.	O	O			O
I interact with my broader community in ways that interest me.	O	O	O	O	O
I am happy and my needs are met in my current romantic and intimate relationships.	O	O	O	O	O
I am content with my family structure and size.	O	O	O	O	O
I feel accepted and included in my social groups.	O	O	O	O	O
I have enough friends to share and pursue interests with.	O	O	O	O	O
I am interested in pursuing new or alternative relationships.	O	O	O	O	O

Professional

	Strongly Disagree				Strongly Agree
I have completed the necessary education to pursue the careers I want.	O	o	o	o	O
All of my professional training requirements are current.	O	o	o	o	O
I have secured the required certifications for my current position.	O	o	o	o	O
I am fully confident in my professional skills.	O	o	o	o	O
I am able to maintain a work-life balance.	O	o	o	o	O
I am interested in pursuing a different career or industry.	O	o	o	o	O
I am interested in pursuing a leadership role within my profession.	O	o	o	o	O
I am interested in sharing my professional skills through teaching or mentoring others.	O	o	o	o	O
I am interested in pursuing a position in a different organization.	O	o	o	o	O

Adventure

	Strongly Disagree				Strongly Agree
I have regularly pursue my hobbies or interests.	O	o	o	o	O
I am satisfied with the amount I have traveled.	O	o	o	o	O
I routinely explore new places.	O	o	o	o	O
I am interested in learning a new skill or craft.	O	o	o	o	O
I am satisfied with how much I read.	O	o	o	o	O
I am interested in exploring new cultures	O	o	o	o	O
I would like to dedicate more time dedicated to creating art or a body of work.	O	o	o	o	O
I would like to learn more about a few topics I find interesting.	O	o	o	o	O
I have completed all the items on my "bucket list".	O	o	o	o	O

Rate your overall satisfaction with your status in each realm of your life.

Overall Ratings	Very Unsatisfied				Very Satisfied
Physical	O	o	o	o	O
Emotional	O	o	o	o	O
Social	O	o	o	o	O
Professional	O	o	o	o	O
Adventure	O	o	o	o	O

What three accomplishments are you most proud of from the last 50-weeks?

1)...
....
2)...
....
3)...
....

As you move forward with your personal development, what three changes would you like to prioritize?

1)...
....
2)...
....
3)...
....

Now it's time to ask yourself; *what kind of person you want to be?*

References

Preparation

1.Locke, E. A., Shaw, K. N., Saari, L. M., & Latham, G. P. (1981). Goal setting and task performance: 1969–1980. Psychological Bulletin, 90(1), 125–152. https://doi.org/10.1037/0033-2909.90.1.125

2. De Haas, M., Algera, J., Van Tuijl, H. & Meulman, J. (2000). Macro and Micro Goal Setting: In Search of Coherence. Applied Psychology, 49: 579-595. https://doi.org/10.1111/1464-0597.00033

3. Doran, G.T. (1981). There's a SMART Way to Write Management's Goals and Objectives. Journal of Management Review, 70, 35-36

Phase 1

4. Kruse, K. (2013). Top 100 Inspirational Quotes. Retrieved from https://www.forbes.com/sites/kevinkruse/2013/05/28/inspirational-quotes/?sh=64e6fd9d6c7a

5. Zipkin, N. (2017). 50 Inspirational Quotes to Help You Achieve Your Goals. Retrieved from https://www.entrepreneur.com/leadership/50-inspirational-quotes-to-help-you-achieve-your-goals/287870.

6. Locke, E. A., Shaw, K. N., Saari, L. M., & Latham, G. P. (1981). Goal setting and task performance: 1969–1980. Psychological Bulletin, 90(1), 125–152. https://doi.org/10.1037/0033-2909.90.1.125

7. Forbes India. (2023). 100+ Motivational quotes to inspire a positive mindset for success in your life. Retrieved from https://www.forbesindia.com/article/explainers/motivational-quotes/84853/1.

8. Goodman, E. (2023). 45 Inspirational Quotes for Women that Empower and Motivate. Retrieved from https://www.rd.com/list/womens-history-quotes/.

9. Hopfner, J., & Keith, N. (2021). Goal Missed, Self Hit: Goal-Setting, Goal-Failure, and Their Affective, Motivational, and Behavioral Consequences. Frontiers in Psychology, 12. https://www.frontiersin.org/articles/10.3389/fpsyg.2021.704790

Phase 2

10. Zipkin, N. (2017). 50 Inspirational Quotes to Help You Achieve Your Goals. Retrieved from https://www.entrepreneur.com/leadership/50-inspirational-quotes-to-help-you-achieve-your-goals/287870.

11. Forbes India. (2023). 100+ Motivational quotes to inspire a positive mindset for success in your life. Retrieved from https://www.forbesindia.com/article/explainers/motivational-quotes/84853/1.

12. Zarrin, S., Gracia, E., & Paizao, M. (2020). Prediction of Academic Procrastination by Fear of Failure and Self-Regulation. Education Sciences: Theory & Practice, 20(3), 34-43. https://files.eric.ed.gov/fulltext/EJ1261814.pdf

13. Goodman, E. (2023). 45 Inspirational Quotes for Women that Empower and Motivate. Retrieved from https://www.rd.com/list/womens-history-quotes/.

14. Kruse, K. (2013). Top 100 Inspirational Quotes. Retrieved from https://www.forbes.com/sites/kevinkruse/2013/05/28/inspirational-quotes/?sh=64e6fd9d6c7a

15. Harkin, B., Webb, T. L., Chang, B. P., Prestwich, A., Conner, M., Kellar, I., Benn, Y., & Sheeran, P. (2016). Does monitoring goal progress promote goal attainment? A meta-analysis of the experimental evidence. Psychological bulletin, 142(2), 198–229. https://doi.org/10.1037/bul0000025

Phase 3

16. Zipkin, N. (2017). 50 Inspirational Quotes to Help You Achieve Your Goals. Retrieved from https://www.entrepreneur.com/leadership/50-inspirational-quotes-to-help-you-achieve-your-goals/287870.

17. Forbes India. (2023). 100+ Motivational quotes to inspire a positive mindset for success in your life. Retrieved from https://www.forbesindia.com/article/explainers/motivational-quotes/84853/1.

18. TD Bank. (2016). Visualizing Goals Influences Financial Health and Happiness, Study Finds. Retrieved from https://stories.td.com/us/en/article/visualizing-goals-influences-financial-health-and-happiness-study-finds.

19. Goodman, E. (2023). 45 Inspirational Quotes for Women that Empower and Motivate. Retrieved from https://www.rd.com/list/womens-history-quotes/.

20. Smith, P. (2023). 30 Greatest Motivational Sports Quotes of All-time. Retrieved from https://marathonhandbook.com/motivational-sports-quotes/ .

21. Malgorzata, M., Nesterak, J., Sołtysik, M., Szymla, W., & Wojnarowska, M,(2020). Multitasking Effects on Individual Performance: An Experimental Eye-Tracking Study, European Research Studies Journal Volume XXIII Issue 1, 107-116.

Phase 4

22. Smith, P. (2023). 30 Greatest Motivational Sports Quotes of All-time. Retrieved from https://marathonhandbook.com/motivational-sports-quotes/ .

23. Goodman, E. (2023). 45 Inspirational Quotes for Women that Empower and Motivate. Retrieved from https://www.rd.com/list/womens-history-quotes/.

24. Gardner, S., & Albee, D. (2015). "Study focuses on strategies for achieving goals, resolutions". Press Releases. 266.

25. Forbes India. (2023). 100+ Motivational quotes to inspire a positive mindset for success in your life. Retrieved from https://www.forbesindia.com/article/explainers/motivational-quotes/84853/1.

26. Zipkin, N. (2017). 50 Inspirational Quotes to Help You Achieve Your Goals. Retrieved from https://www.entrepreneur.com/leadership/50-inspirational-quotes-to-help-you-achieve-your-goals/287870.

27. Mrazek, M. D., Franklin, M. S., Phillips, D. T., Baird, B., & Schooler, J. W. (2013). Mindfulness training improves working memory capacity and GRE performance while reducing mind wandering. Psychological science, 24(5), 776–781. https://doi.org/10.1177/0956797612459659

Phase 5

28. Zipkin, N. (2017). 50 Inspirational Quotes to Help You Achieve Your Goals. Retrieved from https://www.entrepreneur.com/leadership/50-inspirational-quotes-to-help-you-achieve-your-goals/287870.

29. Smith, P. (2023). 30 Greatest Motivational Sports Quotes of All-time. Retrieved from https://marathonhandbook.com/motivational-sports-quotes/ .

30. Gafner, J. (2023). The Self-Advocacy Gap for Women. Retrieved from https://marathonhandbook.com/motivational-sports-quotes/ .

31. Kruse, K. (2013). Top 100 Inspirational Quotes. Retrieved from https://www.forbes.com/sites/kevinkruse/2013/05/28/inspirational-quotes/?sh=64e6fd9d6c7a.

32. Forbes India. (2023). 100+ Motivational quotes to inspire a positive mindset for success in your life. Retrieved from https://www.forbesindia.com/article/explainers/motivational-quotes/84853/1.

33. Gardner, S., & Albee, D. (2015). "Study focuses on strategies for achieving goals, resolutions". Press Releases. 266.

Printed in the USA
CPSIA information can be obtained
at www.ICGtesting.com
LVHW060312181123
764002LV00021B/53